HOW TO CURE HYPERTENSION AND THE EFFECTS IT HAS ON YOUR SEX LIFE USING YOGA

Author: John Richards

Cover image courtesy of: FreeDigitalPhotos.net

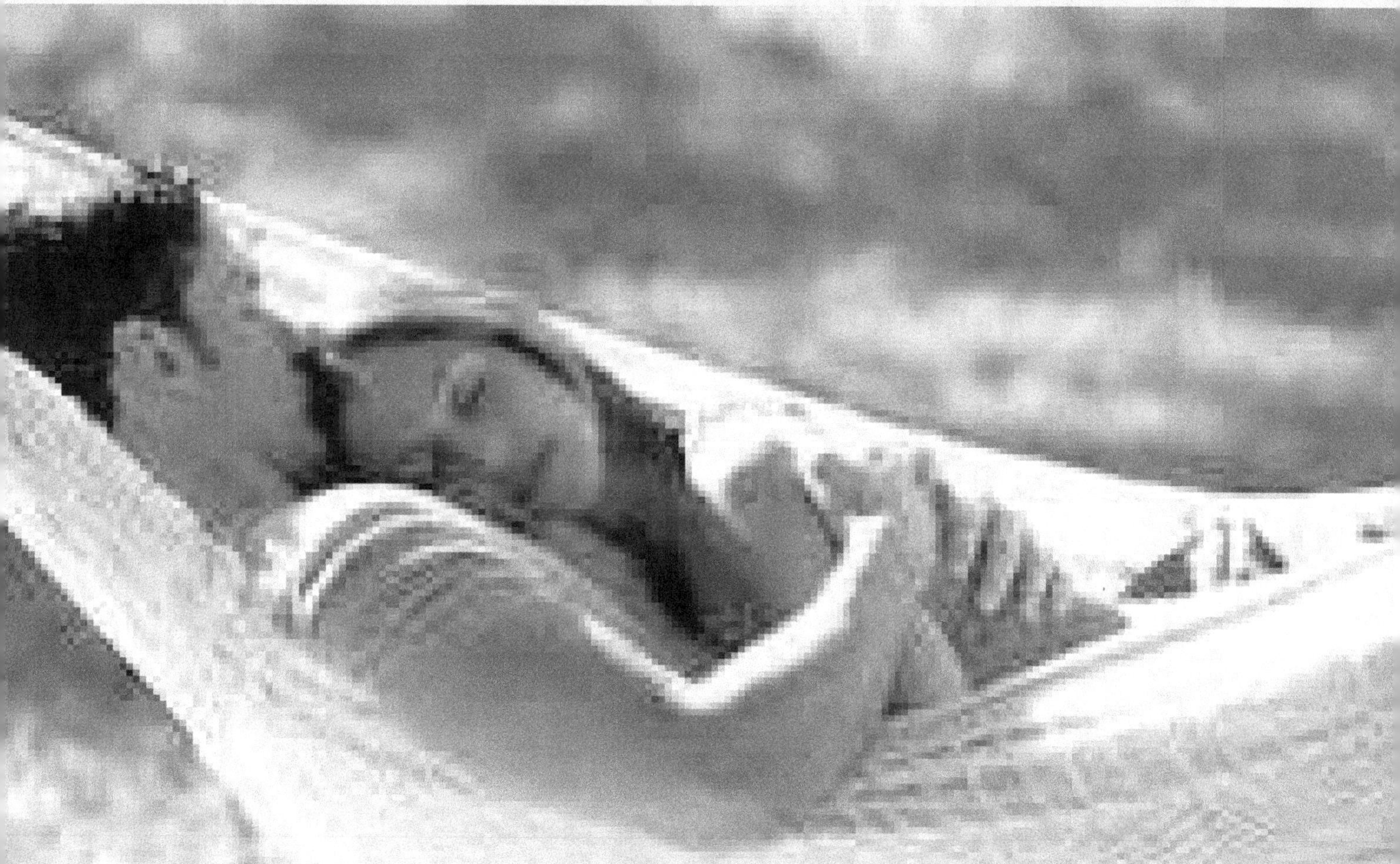

CONTENTS:

Acknowledgement

Introduction

Hypertension

Causes of High Blood Pressure

Anatomy of an Erection

Erectile Dysfunction

Sex Life

Promote Well-Being

Nutrition for High Blood Pressure

L-Arginine Rich Foods

Natural Ways to Cure High Blood Pressure

Best Yoga Poses for High Blood Pressure

Yoga Poses for Better Sex-Drive

Conclusion

Acknowledgement

I would like to thank you for downloading this book, "How to Cure Hypertension And The Effects It Has On Your Sex Life Using Yoga".

This book demonstrates step by step the best techniques to choose to make Yoga a regular part of your life as well as a good nutrition plan to accommodate your yoga routine so you can sustain and empower your body and to have a more energetic, vibrant and magnificent sexual co-existence with your partner!

This is a short and essential book that offers proposals on how you can start to move for brilliant sexual activity along with the natural cures of High Blood Pressure. This book is to make it as uncomplicated as it possibly can.

Yoga exercises with specific postures and legitimate routine can totally bring happiness into your life!

The proposed nutrition for High Blood Pressure can make the healthiest and most delightful dinners. This natural sustenance consuming regimen is about preparing whatever you require, at whatever point you need!

You can get fit as a fiddle, recover your body, and enhance your sex-drive, look and feel more energetic, not in years, not in months but in a short time!

Continuing with Yoga and specific food lifestyle, there's positively no choice of individuals asking "Where do you get your nourishment from?"

There's so much misunderstanding and socially imbued myths about sustenance, on extent, quality and its source and especially about complete vs. insufficient nutrients.

Most people have no idea how a simple combo of cucumber and celery can make a major difference, coupled with protein as they have a good source of amino acids also.

As long as we consume a more plant based regimen, we will be able to get ALL of The required nutrients we need.

This has more than once being demonstrated with the example of top athletes transitioning to plant-based consuming regimens and having enormous accomplishment in their professional games.

It is scientifically proved that consuming a non-vegan based eating regimen will tend to have more harmful effects on your overall well being as opposed to eating vegan.

We simply need something like 5%-10% of our calories to come from protein, and surprisingly enough, this is the extent practically all fruits & vegetables fall into.

Introduction

As the heart beats, it moves blood through the arteries on its route to the rest of the body. Pulse is the measure of pressure made inside the arteries and veins.

Systolic circulatory pressure is measured as the blood pumps out of the heart. Diastolic circulatory pressure is measured between heart-beats. Blood pressure differs from individual to individual and can change for the duration of the day.

Normal Blood pressure is vital for healthy well-being. Typical pulse is 120/80mmhg. At the point when pulse surpasses these values we call it hypertension.

High blood pressure causes imperviousness to the pumping of the blood ± this obliges that the heart work harder than natural to flow blood through the blood vessels and to keep up that raised circulatory pressure.

In the long run this leads towards desperate wellbeing results and life undermining medicinal conditions.

High Blood Pressure doesn't generally show evident manifestations. But it causes dynamic harm to arteries and veins, which can meddle with blood flow all through the body.

This may result stroke, coronary illness, and heart failure. Different parts of the body, including the kidneys, legs, and eyes may likewise endure harm.

The circulatory systems transports oxygenated blood all through the body. Strong arteries extend marginally as blood is pumped through them.

High Blood Pressure may cause the arteries to extend excessively, abandoning them vulnerable to harm. About whether, little tears structure scar tissue inside the arteries.

Any part of the body that doesn't accept enough oxygenated blood is at danger. Ache or numbness may be an indication of impeded blood flow to your limbs, bringing about fringe artery disease. This expands the possibility of contamination or tissue death, such as, gangrene.

Our mind can't work without a continuous supply of oxygenated blood. Contracted arteries or blood coagulation can quickly hinder the flow of blood to the mind.

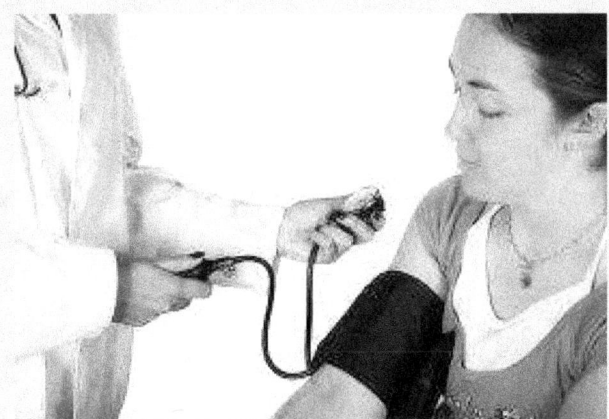

For this situation individuals are at more danger of an out stroke, an incident in which the blood supply to a part of the mind is cut off, and creating cerebrum cells to die.

Stroke can result in extreme, sometimes irreversible harm, contingent upon the part of the mind involved. The greatest danger for stroke is hypertension.

The kidneys filter waste items, keeping what you require, and disposing of what your body can't use. The kidneys can't work without a regular supply of oxygenated blood.

Narrowed veins confine the regular blood supply, bringing on the kidneys to develop less efficient in uprooting toxins. One of the most noteworthy danger causes for kidney failure is high blood pressure.

High Blood Pressure can result in sexual dysfunction in men and women. In men, regular blood flow to the penis is important to accomplish and keep up an erection.

In the event that severe high blood pressure influences arteries and veins leading the penis, it can bring about erectile dysfunction (ED), painful ejaculation, and impotence.

In women, high blood pressure can influence the blood flow to the vagina. That can result in vaginal dryness, painful intercourse, lessened sexual yearning, and inconvenience attaining orgasm.

Sexual dysfunction can result in anxiety in both partners and possibly result in relationship issues.

If by chance your sexual life is all of a sudden losing steam and you're humiliated or stressed over your sexual response, you're surely not alone.

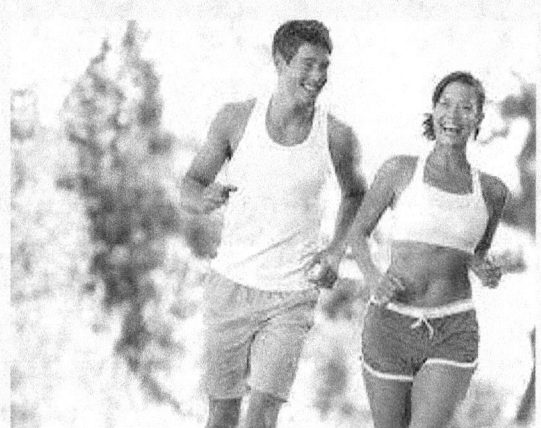

A large number of men and women impart your stress over inconveniences in their sexual life and your stress about satisfying your sexual accomplice. At the same time most have no solution how simple the result might be.

Our skeletal system needs calcium to keep up strong and healthy bones. A part of WKH NLGQH\IV function is to filter urine. At the point when the kidneys don't work appropriately, you may discharge an excessive amount of calcium in the urine.

If insufficient calcium stays available for use for your bones, bone thickness decreases and increasing the danger for osteoporosis. Bones get feeble, fragile, and more prone to cracks and breaks.

Hypertension

High Blood Pressure is simply an increase in blood circulatory pressure, while Hypertension is a disease. Slight expand in pulse is natural in daily life.

Such as when you exercise or walk fast or when you get irate or excited, your heart begins pulsating fast and this raises your circulatory pressure.

That is nothing to stress over, it's a natural process of your body to adapt to your movement or emotions and a part of being sound.

At the point when your circulatory pressure remains constantly raised for a considerable length of time even while you are resting, that is the moment that you ought to begin to worry that it is not beneficial.

If the circulatory pressure remains constantly elevated over the month that implies that you have Hypertension.

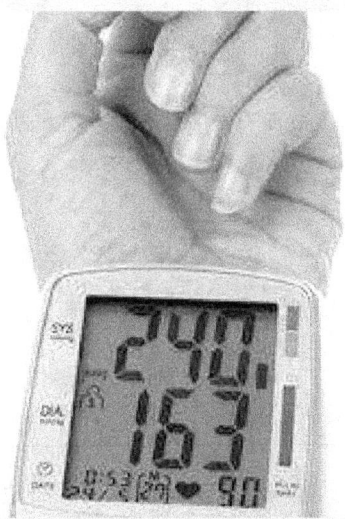

Having hypertension will in fact be a serious problem for you and can Stress you a lot. We will instruct you about hypertension and let you know how to carry on a healthy and effortless life. With strong will and legitimate direction you don't need to stress over high blood pressure ever again.

Hypertension adversely influences your heart as well as harms your kidneys, eyes, blood vessels and cerebrum. These are the real organs of your body, and having hypertension puts your life at danger from harm to these organs.

There are other minor unfavorable impacts too. These provide for us reason enough to be profoundly worried about keeping up our blood pressure in the natural condition ± which would elevate all the pressure on these organs.

Sex is similar to any of the other exercises in the extent that the physical benefits gained from the activity are concerned. It gets the heart pumping; however would it say it is ok for people with heart problem?

One of the most serious issues with hypertension is that some individuals who have it don't feel it. The unknown prompt symptoms make it not entirely obvious, or stop drug medicine when reactions show up.

There is a natural relationship between pulse and sex drive. On one side is the risk that hypertension patients are presented to, and on the other side is the impact that medications for high blood pressure have on sex-act.

Hypertension can influence the sex drive of both men and women. In men, hypertension can result in erectile issues by reducing the flow of blood to the penis.

Hypertensive women are more prone to experience pain during the sex-act because of a noteworthy lessen of lubrication, and they may experience problem in arriving to an orgasm.

Causes of High Blood Pressure

In spite of the fact that High Blood Pressure is a life undermining incident, it can normally go without any signs or indications.

That is the reason it is known as the silent killer, yet indications do happen when your blood pressure gets to be high to the point that your body can't endure it. So many individuals with hypertension report these symptoms:

⌨ Migraines (especially in the back of the head)

- Unsteadiness

- Headache

- Dizziness

- Buzzing or ringing in the ears

- Blurred or altered vision

- Blacking out incidents

The exact reason for hypertension depends from person to person. Factors and conditions causing the progression of hypertension are:

- Smoking

- Over Weight or Obesity

- Lack of physical movements

- Stationary lifestyle

- Intake of More Salt

- High Alcohol Intake

- Old Age

- Heredity

- Prolonged Kidney Infection

- Adrenal and Thyroid Issues

- Drugs that restrict Blood Vessels

- High Cholesterol

- Narrowing of Arteries because of more lipid content in the Body

- Stress

- Pregnancy

- Birth Control pills (particularly those containing Estrogen)

The sexual ability has a scientific connection between hormones, neurotransmitters (dopamine and serotonin), and the sexual organs.

While dopamine improves, serotonin represses sexual capacity. As drugs treat by pushing or controlling specific reactions in the body, they can influence sex drive and performance.

Medicines of Blood Pressure that meddle with the secretion of testosterone essential for arousal are prone to diminish sex drive. Erection is accomplished after an essential coordination between nerves, hormones, veins and psychological situations.

Ejaculation is a complex reflex activity incorporating the enactment of alpha-receptors in the prostate organ and seminal liquid.

During discharge, the bladder neck is closed to permit the semen to flow out of through the penis. Drugs that meddle with this process lead to ejaculatory hindrances like failure to discharge.

Heredity positively assumes a real part in your pulse rate, yet that doesn't mean your destiny is fixed if your dad had the condition.

Regardless of the possibility that you have the hereditary reason, you may have the capacity to override it by heading a dynamic and magnificent lifestyle.

Anxiety expands your pulse for a short period and when it is diminished your blood pressure strain comes back to normal.

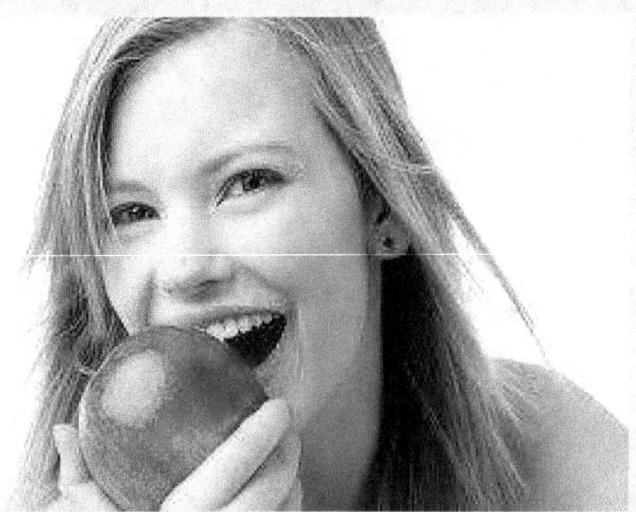

Stress has not been given reason to really cause hypertension. However if you are leading a disturbed and stressful life, for short periods, you may observe that you are not consuming a healthy eating regimen, smoking or drinking an excess of and not taking enough physical work out.

All these things will enhance raising your blood pressure.

Beyond any doubt being focused on reasons our blood pressure to rise for a couple of minutes.

When we feel stressed our bodies discharge adrenaline and our heart rates and blood pressure rise as our body get settled for some activity. But this impact just keeps up a couple of minutes and after that our blood pressure comes back to normal.

Conversely, real hypertension is having for all time raised level for weeks, months and years. As such, it has not been demonstrated that customary short release of adrenaline instigated blood pressure rises have any enduring impact on the body.

Actually the rates of hypertension and coronary illness are the same among individuals who don't have distressing job as compared to the individuals with anxiety filled occupations.

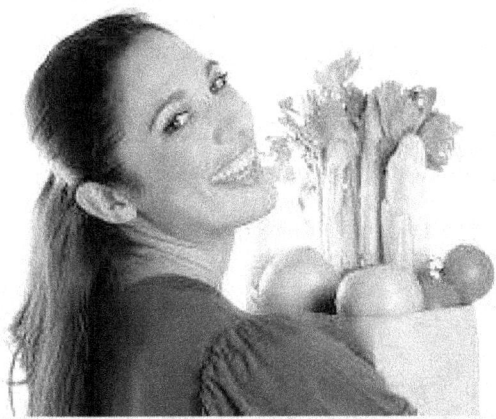

People may deal with stress in the ways that may enhance their danger of hypertension.

They may consume processed foods that are high in salt, neglect to consume enough fruits and vegetables, smoke or drink a lot of alcohol. They might also strive to give time to be dynamic with routine physical exercises.

Without a doubt more individuals have heart attacks in the winter than in the sunny season. Low temperatures make our blood vessels contract to conserve high temperature and keep up body temperature.

This implies that there is less space for our blood to flow in, increasing the blood pressure and heart rate, and thickening the blood.

On the off chance that you have contracted arteries, these elements may cause chest torments and increase the probability of blood clumps framing in the blood vessels, which can prompt a heart attack.

The danger of this occurrence is more in individuals with hypertension. The best guidance is to abstain from being exposed to the cold for long time and to wrap up warm clothes.

Anatomy of an Erection

An erection is the result of balanced coordination between nerves, hormones, blood vessels and psychological situations.

Medicines that have a physical impact on the blood vessels in the penis, those that follow up on the mental stimulation or meddle with hormone levels (especially testosterone) or influence the transmission of nerve messages, can all reason impotence.

Hypertension is likewise known factor variable for affecting erectile dysfunction.

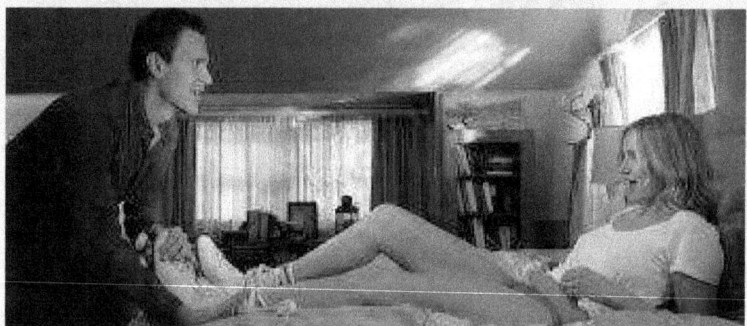

Hypertension that is not appropriately controlled is going to debilitate your body's capability to enhance blood flow when required, making it more troublesome for you to accomplish an erection.

In the pole of the penis there are two adjoining chambers of corpora spongy tissues. They're essentially responsible for erections. Another chamber Corpus spongy is just below them. The urethra, which brings semen and urine, goes through the core of it.

The corpora spongy tissues are made of small blood vessels, smooth muscle fiber, and unfilled spaces. The chambers are wrapped in a cover of thin tissues.

When you get an erection, signals from the neurons in the penis cause the smooth muscle of the chambers to unwind and blood vessels to enlarge, or open larger. This permits a surge of blood to fill the unfilled spaces.

The blood pressure flow causes the cover of tissues around the chambers press on blood vessels that ordinarily empty blood out from the penis. That holds blood in the penis. As more blood flows in, the penis grows and hardened, and you have an erection.

At the point when the excitement finishes, the smooth muscles contract again, taking pressure off the blood vessels and permitting blood to flow back out from the penis. Lastly the penis comes back to a loose state.

Erectile Dysfunction

Hypertension can meddle with a fulfilling sexual act as it can change blood circulation patterns in the body and harm the inner surface of blood vessels, both of which may lessen blood flow to the penis and vagina.

Hypertension is a significant reason for erection issues. Hypertension keeps the supply routes that convey blood into the penis from widening the way it should be.

It likewise makes the smooth muscle in the penis lose its capacity to unwind. Therefore, insufficient blood flows into the penis to make it erect.

Men with hypertension might also have a low testosterone level. Testosterone is the male hormone that functions a big part in sexual arousal.

Hypertension without any other input can prompt erectile dysfunction. Yet a few medications for treating hypertension can be the reason also.

At times, the harmful addictions that some men with hypertension make can add to the issue. Such as, smoking builds circulatory pressure, and harms the blood vessels and decreases blood flow all around the body.

To treat erectile dysfunction, one must bring down the blood pressure if its high. Some individuals can do that through lifestyle changes alone. Others need help from medicines of high blood pressure.

An issue for some men is that a few sorts of hypertension prescriptions can also cause erectile dysfunction. That may make it hard to continue on your prescription, particularly if your hypertension never brought about any symptoms before.

Hypertension usually has no signs or side effects. At the same time the effect on your sexual life to be self-evident. Naturally sexual action is unrealistic to represent a prompt risk to your wellbeing, such as; a heart attack and hypertension can influence your normal fulfillment with sex.

A connection between hypertension and sexual issues can have major un-wanted results in men.

.

Sex Life

As per numerous researches, hypertension is affected by the anxiety and strain of an advanced lifestyle.

The research that recommends regular yogic practices and diet regimen can help to enhance wellbeing and mental prosperity, enhancing flexibility to stress and also to hypertension.

It may appear as though expressing the self-evident, yet if one controls stress on the brain and the body by consuming healthy eating plan centered on pure, fresh, wholesome and nutritious diet, practicing yoga postures. *Natural activities such as Pranayama* and meditation can greatly control high blood pressure.

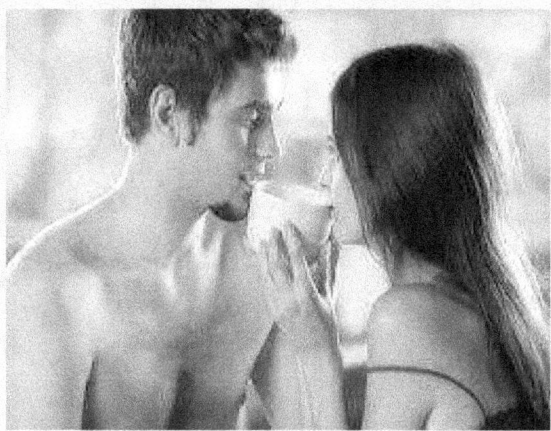

You may over think how sex can influence your blood pressure, or if it is secure to have intercourse whatsoever.

These reasons of fear are natural so it could be consoling to realize that sex, in the same way as any activity, raises your blood pressure yet for a short time. Your blood pressure falls promptly within a short time. This provisional build in blood pressure is natural and safe.

Sex ought to be considered an optional type of physical movement, no more unpleasant to the heart than different types of moderate exercises.

In some cases hypertension, and HBP bringing down medications, can result in issues with sex.

Some men may have issues with weakness or impotence. A ratio of the physical reasons for impotence incorporates hypertension and coronary illness. Prolonged hypertension can influence the blood vessels in the penis, making it harder to have an erection.

Weakness or impotence can likewise happen as a symptom of HBP bringing down pills, specifically **diuretics** and **beta blockers**. Impotence that is created by medications is normally reversible.

Hypertension can lessen blood flow to the vagina. Women might every so often find that sex is unpleasant and tormenting or that they are not interested to have a climax.

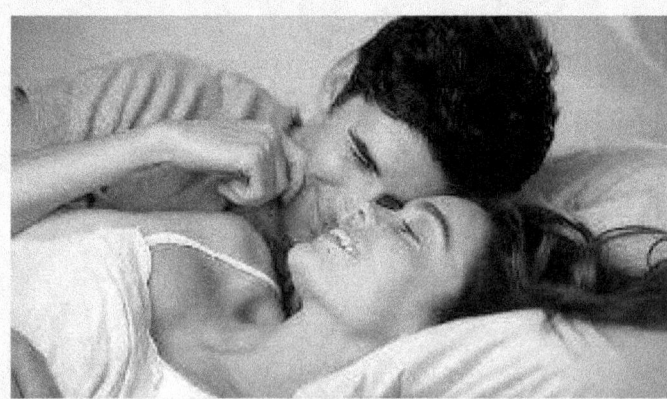

Hypertension itself does not result in loss of sexual longing. In any case if you are concerned over your wellbeing you may observe that you would prefer not to engage in sexual relations.

Try to discuss with your accomplice about how you are feeling; its not difficult to feel rejected when sexual closeness changes.

Holding closeness within your relationship will help to overcome challenges. Keep in mind that you can express your emotions in many distinctive ways, for instance through talking, with non-verbal communication and physical contact, such as, kissing and nestling.

Seldom heart attacks can happen in between sexual act period. This is comparatively unique with different exercises which raise your blood pressure for similar periods of time.

Capacity for Men

In men, the reduced blood flow can decrease sexual longing and meddle with erections and discharge.

Hypertension harms the covering of the blood vessels and reasons them to harden and slender, restricting blood flow. This results less blood flow to the penis.

For some men, the reduced blood flow makes it hard to accomplish and keep up erections and it is termed to as erectile dysfunction. The issue is reasonably basic, particularly among men who are not treating their hypertension.

Indeed a single incident of erectile dysfunction can result in tension. Expects that it will happen again may lead men to disregard sex act and it influences association with their sexual accomplice.

Hypertension can likewise meddle with discharge and diminish sexual craving. Once in a while the drugs used to treat hypertension have same impacts.

Capacity for Women

Hypertension impact on sexual issues in women isn't well confirmed. Anyway its probable that hypertension could influence a woman's sexual life.

In women, it can prompt vaginal dryness, a diminishing in sexual longing, and troubles accomplishing climax.

Hypertension can lessen blood flow to the vagina. For some women, this prompts a reduction in sexual longing or arousal, vaginal dryness, or trouble attaining climax. Enhancing arousal, foreplay and lubrication can offer assistance. Like men, ladies can also experience anxiety, uneasiness and relationship issues because of sexual dysfunction.

Promote Well-Being

By managing on healthy lifestyle options, you can bring down your HBP and conceivably enhance your sexual life.

If you are overweight, losing your weight around eating regimen and specific aerobic or Yoga exercises might be an exceptionally viable approach to bring down your blood pressure.

Other dietary controls can additionally be useful. These incorporate having a high-fiber, low fat diet and low sugar diet. Evading more liquor consumption can additionally be useful. For a low salt eating regimen to bring down your blood pressure your salt inclusion must be up to sustainable requirement.

Slimming down the body brings down blood pressure in most individuals. Truth to be told, for each one pound lost, blood pressure may drop by two points.

Shedding pounds may help you reduce the measure of medicine you take or even get you off drug totally. Indeed a little measure of weight loss is helpful.

Managing nutritional insufficiencies can likewise be very useful in bringing down hypertension. Utilizing nutritious supplements with the below suggestions could be especially useful:

- Take a sufficient vitamin supplement to get ideal levels of vitamins A, C, and D in addition to magnesium.

- Intake of Calcium 700-900 mg every day!

- Potassium- The measure of potassium found in one banana and 1 glass of tomato juice a day can likewise help to reduce blood pressure.

- Coenzyme Q10 200 milligrams a day can additionally be exceptionally compelling. Coenzyme Q10 lack is common in individuals taking cholesterol-control drugs.

- Dark chocolate- In spite of the fact that it just brings down blood pressure by 3-4 mm, it tastes great and is rich in antioxidants.

Dietary and lifestyle progressions can enhance HBP control and reduce the danger of charted wellbeing issues. While HBP medicine is essential for the individuals, for whom lifestyle progressions are inadequate or ineffective.

Lifestyle changes suggestions for the individuals with High Blood Pressure:

- Weight Loss- Keep up a normal weight with a target Body Mass Index of 18 to 25.

- DASH Diet arrangement- Adopt an eating regimen rich in fruits, vegetables, and low-fat dairy items. Decrease the consumption of saturated fats.

- Lower Salt Intake- Decrease the salt intake to a measure of one teaspoon a day.

- Yoga or Aerobic Physical Activity- Manage to start the brisk morning walking for at least 30 minutes per day along with specific Yoga postures.

▣ Balance of Alcohol Consumption- Men should limit liquor consumption to two drinks for every day. Constraining the measure of liquor to 2 drinks is relied upon to bring down blood pressure. This likewise ensures your liver and kidneys from harm.

Obviously, a leaner body can support your certainty and help you feel more splendid, which could likewise enhance your sexual life.

Your sexual stimulation may shift with emotions about your accomplice and the situations in which sex happens. To energize fulfilling sex, begin sex act when you and your accomplice are feeling relaxed.

Try to explore different approaches to be physically cozy, such as, massage, foreplay or affectionate behavior. Offer with one another the sorts of specific sexual actions you revel in most. You may find that open sharing talks are the most ideal approach to accomplish sexual fulfillment.

Nutrition for High Blood Pressure

Eating regimen can have immense impact on hypertension. The customary yogic eating regimen is vegan. It is focused around whole grains, fresh fruits and non-vegetarian items aside from milk, yogurt and cheeses.

The human digestive system functions best on a veggie lover diet. Veggie lovers are also less inclined to experience the ill effects of hypertension.

The sustenance you consume can basically influence your blood science and pulse rate. Luckily, an eating plan that is useful for your heart doesn't need to be suffering for your taste buds.

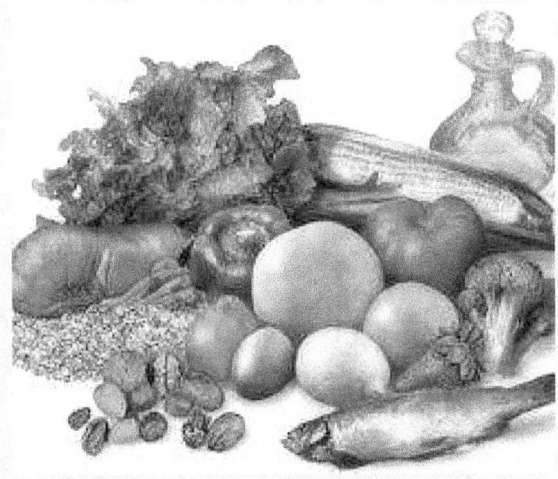

Here are a few recommendations for managing on the right sustenance options for Hypertension:

The consuming arrangement, known as the **DASH Eating Plan** is low in saturated fat, cholesterol, and treats fresh fruits, vegetables, and low-fat dairy sustenance. It also incorporates whole grain items, fish, poultry, and nuts, and it limits meat, desserts, and sugary drinks.

This makes for an eating regimen rich in magnesium, potassium, and calcium, and in addition protein and fiber - a winning composition for bringing down blood pressure.

Reduce Salt-food Consumption- Research utilizing the DASH eating plan and distinctive levels of dietary salt affirmed what has been prompted for a long time ± decreasing dietary salt can help lower pulse rate.

Being touchy to salt implies you tend to hold liquid when you take in more amount of salt, most likely on account of an imperfection in your kidneys' capability to dispose of sodium.

Your body tries to weaken the sodium in the blood by conserving fluids. This constrains your blood vessels to work hard to flow the extra blood volume.

Increase the Potassium intake- Some individuals who have hypertension take diuretics that cause a loss of potassium, so they are advised to consume a banana every day to replace it. Anyhow experts now think more potassium may be a decent thought for everybody.

Not just do we consume an excessive amount of salt, we take in very little potassium. It's the harmony in the middle of sodium and potassium that is thought to be essential to blood pressure.

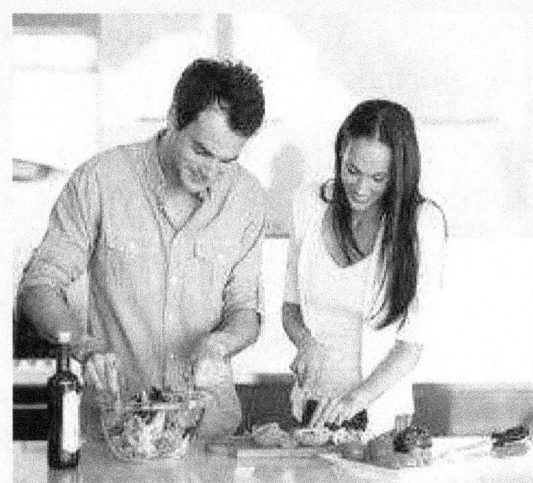

Don't purchase potassium supplements as that could be risky. Both excess of and little potassium can enhance a heart attack. Maintain the nourishment high in potassium to be secured; sustenance rich in potassium incorporate bananas, oranges, potatoes, tomatoes, and milk.

Take more calcium- Your heart needs calcium to keep up its legitimate heart-beat, and your kidneys need calcium to manage your body's sodium: water parity. Research has demonstrated that individuals who have hypertension normally don't get enough dietary calcium.

Different studies affirm that more calcium can result to lower blood pressure. In any case that result is not so much seen with calcium supplements. Depend, rather, on sustenance that is rich in calcium.

Vitamin C- It is an antioxidant and C helps keep free radicals away from harming interior surface of blood vessels, and it may help reduce blood pressure. Take its supplement or consume vitamin C-rich sustenance.

Priority for Garlic- Numerous scientists have indicated garlic's capability to lower pulse rate. It likewise makes an astounding flavor substitution when you're reducing salt in your diet.

Garlic enhances the incredible properties that help you get blood pressure in control. It is possible that raw or cooked garlic helps you in lessening cholesterol level.

When you have your pulse level high then take at consuming 1 or 2 slightly pulverized cloves of garlic naturally. As smashed garlic cloves produce hydrogen sulfide, which helps in enhancing good flow of blood, reduces the pressure on the heart and disposes of gas.

You can likewise take 5 to 6 drops of garlic juice blended with 4 teaspoons of water two times each day for better comes about.

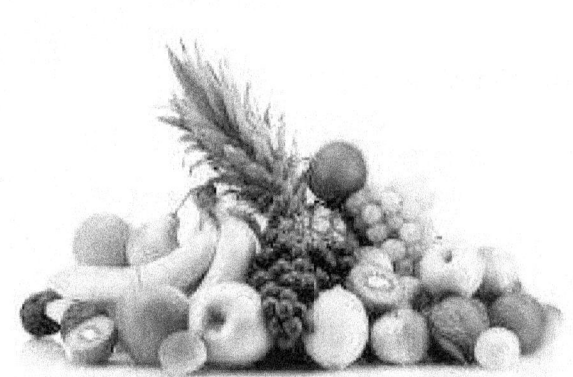

Let Fruits and Vegetables rule- Vegetarians have a much lower ratio of hypertension. You, as well, can benefit from this plan without turning into a veggie lover. Slowly increase your every day servings by sneaking in an additional serving or two at every supper.

You will probably be consuming less fat, more fiber, less salt, and more potassium - and you'll presumably get in shape. Those benefits will help bring down your pulse rate.

You don't need to cut the espresso coffee- Caffeine does not concern of being connected with hypertension.

While it can raise your blood pressure briefly, your body adjusts to the stimulant level if you routinely drink a certain measure of espresso, tea, or cola consistently, and your pulse is no more influenced by these beverages.

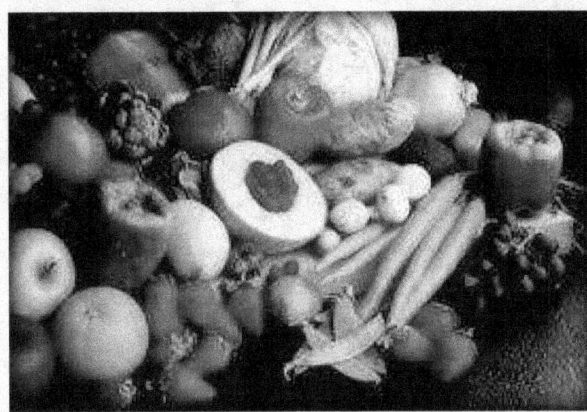

These regular foods are presumably in your kitchen, and all can assume a part as a home solution for control your pulse down.

Bananas- Banana is the best natural solution for blood pressure. Consume one or two bananas every day to keep your hypertension in control. The high potassium in the banana will help you control the blood pressure level. It supports you to be free of cholesterol, with its low sodium levels.

An individual needs three to four servings of potassium rich fruits and vegetables every day. A few experts think adding this sum may benefit for your pulse rate.

If bananas aren't your most loved group of fruit, try to take dried apricots, raisins, currants, orange, and spinach, boiled potato, melon, zucchini and cantaloupe.

Pomegranate Seeds- These are stuffed with vitamin C with antioxidants and are great at helping you keep up a healthy blood circulation during aerobic or Yoga exercise regimen, as per scientists at **Penn State Hershey Heart and Vascular Institute**.

That is on account of low levels of antioxidants in your body can enhance a spike in pulse rate, yet the antioxidants found in pomegranates decrease the increase in blood pressure, prompting a healthier workout and capacity to support routine exercises to burn more calories.

Canola, Mustard seed, or Safflower Oils- Changing to poly-unsaturated oils can have an enormous effect in your blood pressure. Shifting to them will additionally decrease your blood cholesterol level.

Broccoli- This vegetable is high in fiber, and a high fiber eating plan is known to help diminish pulse rate. So include this and other fruits and vegetables that are high in fiber.

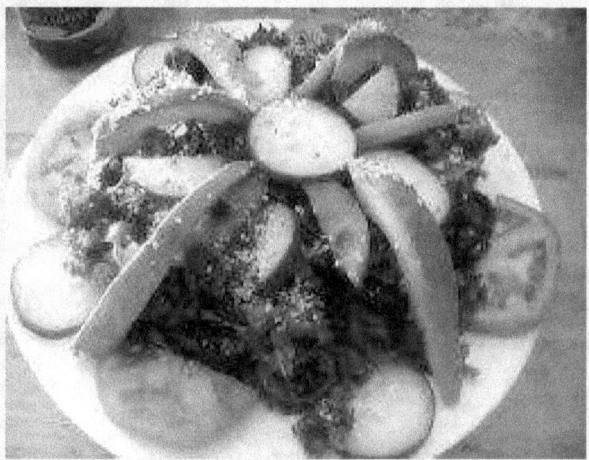

Celery- Since it contains high amounts of nutrients that help lower pulse rate, celery is in a class without any doubt. This supplement is not found in most different vegetables.

Celery might likewise lessen stress hormones that constrict smooth blood flow, so it may be best in those whose hypertension is the consequence of mental anxiety.

Celery contains high amounts of supplement that helps you to control hypertension level. Consume celery consistently to see change in your HBP level. It also helps you in stress hormones decrease that contracts the veins, which may prompt high BP.

If you like celery then you can crunch on to bring down your BP or you can use one stalk of it along with one glass of water daily.

Lemon- Lemon is one of the best solutions for hypertension. It makes the blood vessels delicate and adaptable improving its flexibility, making the pulse levels low. Lemon holds high measures of Vitamin B, so consistently consuming lemon helps you avert for heart problems.

If you are having hypertension then you must drink fresh lemon squeeze many times as could be possible. Drinking one glass lemon juice along with warm water each morning on unfilled stomach is useful for wellbeing. Abstain from including salt or sugar for the desired results.

Nectar Honey- It has a calming impact on your blood vessels and helps in lessening the pressure on the heart, thusly brings down blood pressure.

Devouring 1 or 2 tsp of nectar every day will help you in controlling hypertension. Taking two teaspoons of nectar in the morning on empty stomach is a decent choice.

You can also blend 1 tsp of nectar; 1 tsp of ginger juice and 2 teaspoons of cumin seeds and consume it two times daily. You can likewise consume the mixture of nectar and basil juice on empty stomach for better comes about.

Onion- Onion is a successful solution for bringing down the blood pressure level. You can consume one raw onion (medium) consistently or devour the mixture of nectar and onion juice. Taking 1/2 teaspoon of onion juice blended with 1/2 teaspoon nectar twice consistently will help you in decreasing the blood pressure level. You can perceive a decent change in your BP levels by taking onion squeeze twice a day for about two weeks.

Cayenne Pepper- This red hot spice is a prominent home medicine for mild HBP. If you are experiencing mild hypertension then cayenne pepper is the best regular cure you can take. It makes the blood flow smooth by keeping the blood platelets from becoming clumps and keeps their gathering in the blood.

Cayenne pepper might be added to vegetable salads or fruit salads. You can even include a little cayenne pepper powder into your soup and beverage it. Utilize just a little of cayenne pepper as it is very zesty.

Coconut Water- It is essentially great to keep your body decently hydrated and it is proposed in case you're enduring with HBP. Drink about 8 ± 10 glasses of water daily. You can likewise drink coconut water, along with the water for great results. Coconut water is delicious and possesses nutritional contents too.

They help in bringing down and controlling the HBP levels. You can balance blood pressure level by expending coconut water regularly. You can likewise have a go at utilizing coconut oil rather than other vegetable oils for cooking.

Fenugreek Seeds- These are best solution for bringing down the HBP level. Take one to two teaspoons of fenugreek seeds and boil them in water. Now drain out the water from the fenugreek seeds and bled them in fine glue.

Consume one tablespoon of this glue in the morning on empty stomach and at night regularly. Proceed for a few months to control and bring down your high pulse level.

Consuming one cup of cooked beans, chickpeas, and lentils and legumes as your breakfast can diminish the danger of coronary illness and enhance control of pulse rate.

Watermelon Seeds- Nutrients that are available in Watermelon seeds extend the flexibility of blood vessels. It likewise enhances the kidneys function ability. It also lessens pulse level in joint pain. Take 2 table spoons of dried watermelon seeds (powder) and add them to one mug of boiled water. Leave it for 60 minutes, strain the residue and take 4 tsp of this water at regular interims.

Low Fat Milk- The calcium in milk accomplishes more than assembles strong bones; it assumes an unobtrusive part in forestalling hypertension. Make certain to drink skim milk or consume low fat yogurt. Fresh green vegetables also give calcium.

You ought to do all that you can at home to maintain your HBP down. Along with these home cures, make sure your specialist monitors your condition customarily.

L-Arginine Rich Foods

L-Arginine is an amino acid that is imperatively vital for overall good wellbeing and may be a powerful weapon in the fight against hypertension. Other than assuming a positive part in pulse rate control, arginine can likewise be useful in an assortment of other conditions, including type-2 diabetes and sexual dysfunction in both men and women.

Nitric oxide enters and crosses the membranes of all cells in the body, and it aides manage numerous cell functions. It is even helpful in neurons for the memory capacity.

In blood vessels, Nitric oxide is indispensably essential as it controls the tone of the endothelium, the layer of smooth cells that line the inner surface of blood vessels. If these endothelial cells get non-functional, they can result in constriction influences of blood flow in the vessels that can then prompt hypertension.

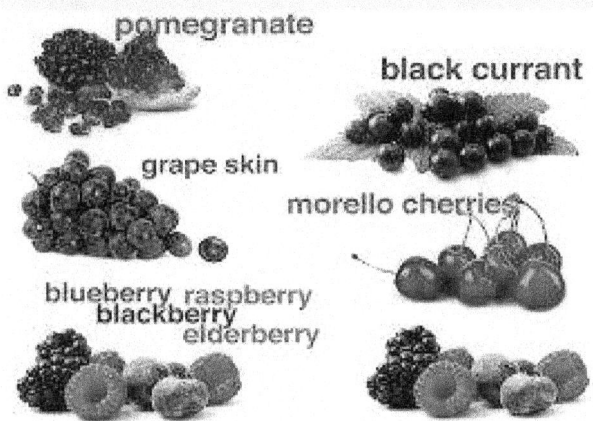

Other than serving to control hypertension, arginine can also give a support to one's sexual coexistence. Nitric oxide released from arginine builds blood flow to the penis in men and to the clitoris in women.

In light of this, men who take arginine regularly have stronger, firmer erections, while women can increase expanded clitoral sensitivity. When you assemble these two, you can see why nearly all real sexual supplements available today contain a big measure of arginine.

- Seafood- Fish is among the highest point of the Arginine nourishment. Different types of fish like, crabs, tuna, squid, lobster, haddock, and salmon are great sources of Arginine. The Salmon is best source of arginine which helps in the relaxation of blood vessels.

- Meat- Along with the proteins, meat additionally contains Arginine. Meats like hamburger, pork, liver, turkey and chicken are known to have Arginine. The liver of these meats contain numerous vitamins, minerals, and arginine. Veal liver is the best source of arginine.

- Eggs- Eggs yolks contain Arginine and it is effortlessly accessible at anybody's home and is liked by all.

- Lentils- Vegetables like peas, peanuts, sunflower seeds, kidney beans, nutty spread, and lima beans have great proportion of Arginine. Nuts and beans are also a source of protein.

⊞ Dark Chocolate- Unsweetened cocoa or hot chocolates are likewise high in Arginine levels.

⊞ Vegetables- Vegetables like soybean, spinach, garlic, mushroom, sea-growth, chives, onion, shallot, peppers, and leeks which are effortlessly accessible help in formation of Arginine. This help to enhance level of Arginine in the body. Soy proteins are exceptionally rich source of arginine.

⊞ Fruits- Fruits are another source of arginine. Fruits have antioxidants, vitamins, minerals with arginine, which is very helpful for human body. Fruits that help in generating Arginine are avocado, grapes, kiwi, strawberry, and watermelon.

⊞ Nuts- Peanuts, almonds, cashew nuts, pistachios, pine-nuts, hazel nuts and walnuts are other sources of Arginine. Their use in diet can also give iron to the body. These nuts additionally have good measure of omega-3 unsaturated fats which serves to keep up healthy skin and hair.

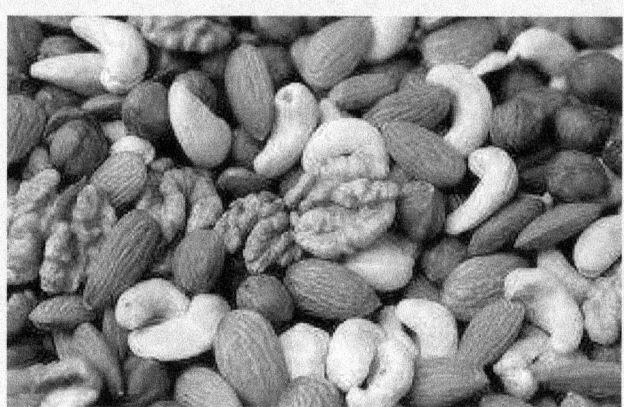

⊞ Grains- Breads and pastas prepared using whole grain wheat are rich in arginine. Whole wheat contains more amount of arginine.

⊞ Drinks- Drinks like black tea, green tea, cocoa, espresso coffee, wine and beer have a little measure of arginine present in them. As such they can satisfy body's necessity of Arginine, however must be taken in little amount due to the presence of caffeine in it.

⊞

Natural Ways to Cure High Blood Pressure

In some cases individuals have a low sex drive without acknowledging they have hypertension. That is the reason it is suggested to get general check-ups to verify there are not any underlying issues.

Some individuals who know they have hypertension may associate it with a lessened sex drive.   Meanwhile, there are many options to treating hypertension without lowering your sex drive.

If you are taking medicine, you can make natural cures to control hypertension and restore your dynamic sexual coexistence.

That incorporates consuming healthy diet, keeping up a healthy weight, routine Yoga or Aerobics, controlling liquor, overseeing stress and practicing relaxation or deep Yoga breathing methods of specific Yoga postures.

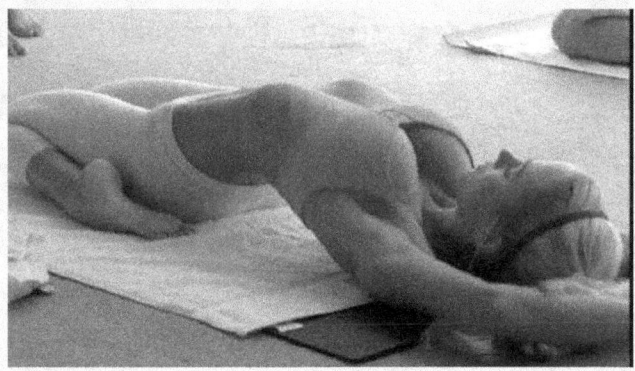

Yoga or Aerobic exercises bring down pulse rate and help you get in shape. If your pulse is high, your specialist may need to get it under control before you start a Yoga or Aerobic activity regimen. This is particularly imperative in the event that you have been inactive.

You ought to be doing exercise activity which keeps you moving/dynamic and makes you inhale more air (Yoga or Aerobic) e.g. brisk walking, swimming, cycling, dancing, running and specific Yoga postures.

You ought to evade any type of practice that includes staying in one spot and forcing to lift, e.g. weight lifting. This is the static activity and it strains your heart and will raise your pulse.

Best Yoga Poses for High Blood Pressure

Keeping up a yoga practice could be a unique approach to diminish anxiety; stays fit as a fiddle and cool the mind.

In any case regarding anxiety easing, not all yoga postures are made equivalent: Some positions are especially viable for enhancing relaxation, stress relief and peacefulness.

Yoga could be a very gainful help to lower hypertension naturally. A tender, calming practice of yoga extends calms brain and body and decreases stress.

Practiced effectively, yoga could be a unique treatment for hypertension. In any case, there are a few suggestions that need to be considered for specific Yoga postures that can help to reduce hypertension.

Regular routine practice of yoga benefits for regulating High Blood Pressure:

- It enhances digestion, blood circulation and immunity

- It improves the functions of nervous system and endocrine organs

- It relaxes body, mind and emotions

- It Controls HBP

- Cures depression, stress and uneasiness

- Enhances blood circulation in the body

- Lessens heart issues like heart attack and chest pain

- Fortifies the brain functioning

- Cures sleep deprivation (Insomnia)

- Removes toxins from the body

- Serves to control anger

- Supplies more oxygen and required blood to all organs of the body

- It serves to manage your routine lifestyle

- Enhances positive thinking

- Enhances immune system to resist for the diseases

- Enhances the ability for the concentration

In Yoga postures the need for blood and oxygen reduces as there are not strains and each muscle is loose.

When done with conscious breathing postures, it balances nervous system bringing about the regulation of blood pressure.

Calming helpful yoga poses are essential for decreasing stress and bringing down blood pressure naturally, as are extending postures like stretching of legs and hip openers.

Support yoga postures that put the spine in an erect position, which permits the heart beat to slow down, as it requires less exertion to pump the blood to the mind.

The Yoga poses that manage the HBP are suitable in with the forward bends, supine, erect sitting, and a few of the reversal postures.

However forward twists are the basic postures to be practiced by persons experiencing hypertension, as the sense organs: eyes, nose, and throat are loose in these postures relaxing the nervous system and making a positive impact on the parasympathetic system.

The below mentioned Yoga postures are beneficial for people suffering from hypertension:

Balasana- Child Pose

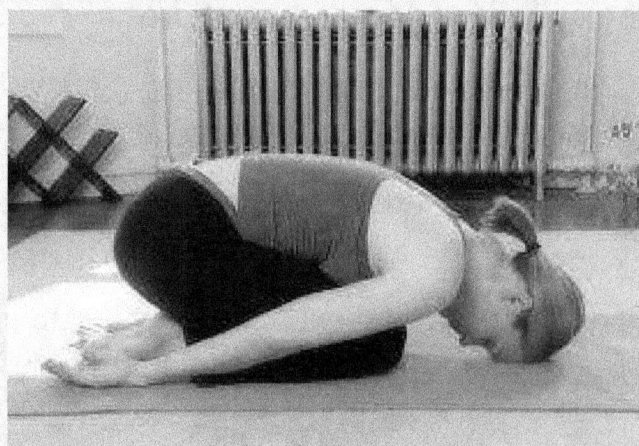

Balasana permits us a chance to inhale completely into the torso of the body. Envision your spine extending and enlarging with every inward breath.

As you breathe out, feel deeper into relaxation, permitting the stretch to discharge mental tension with every breath. Be aware on your breathing to enhance concentration and close out thoughts diversions.

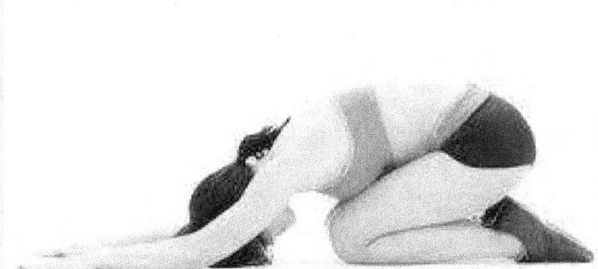

Avoid this Child posture if you have the diarrhea or who are pregnant.

- Releases stress in the back, shoulders and chest midsection

- Recommended if you have dizziness or weariness

- Helps ease anxiety and tension

- Flexes the body's inner organs and keeps them flexible

- Stretches and extends the backbone

- Relieves neck and lower back pain

- It tenderly extends the hips, thighs and lower legs

- Normalizes blood flow all through the body

- Extends muscles, tendons and ligaments in the knee

- Calms the brain and body

- Encourages deep and steady breathing

Padmasana- Lotus Pose

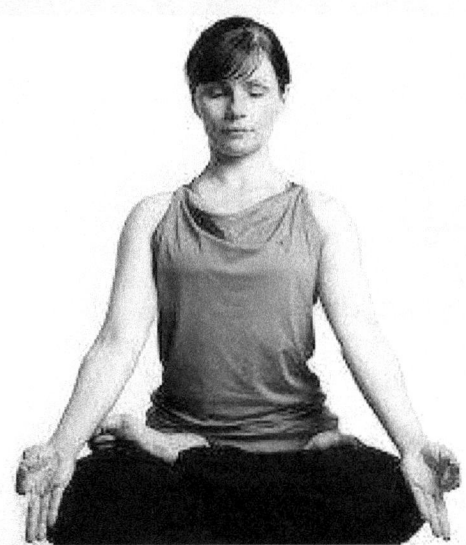

Lotus Pose is sitting traverse leg with the erect spine, making it perfect for meditation and concentration. Make a point to alternate bringing your right and left legs in first.

Steady practice of this posture during the pregnancy is said to help simplify the pains of labor.

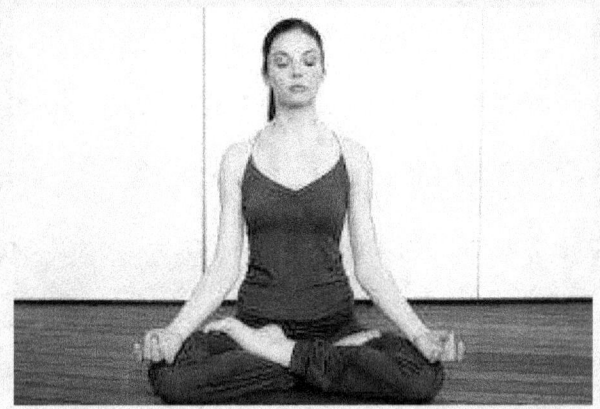

⚏ Opens up the hips portion

⚏ Stretches the lower legs and knees

⚏ calms the mind

⚏ Increases mindfulness and concentration

⚏ Keeps the spine erect

⚏ Helps create good posture

⚏ Eases menstrual issues and sciatica

⚏ Helps keeps all the joints flexible

⚏ Activates the spine, stomach, pelvis, and bladder

⚏ Restores natural vitality levels

Halasana- Plow Pose

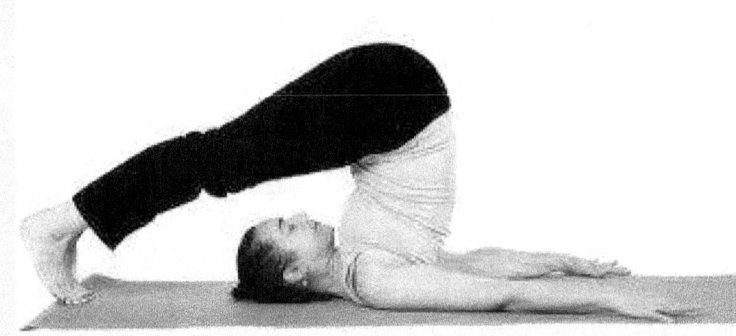

Do this gradually and tenderly. Keep on breathing consistently and supporting your hips your hands, lift them off the ground. Make sure that you don't strain your neck or pressurize it into the ground. Hold this posture and let your body relax more with each consistent breath.

After around a minute of resting in this posture, you might tenderly bring the legs down with exhalation.

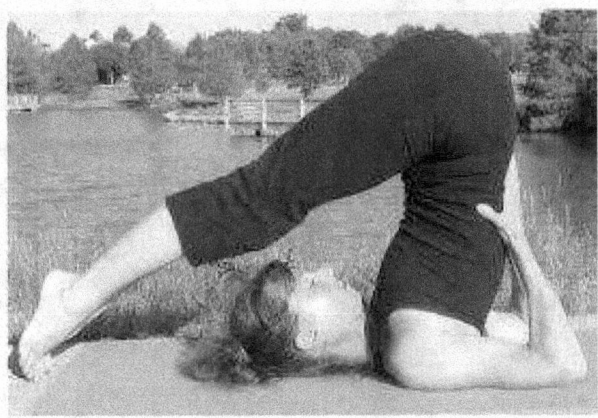

🔲 Strengthens and opens up the neck, shoulders, stomach and back muscles

🔲 Calms the sensory system, lessens stress and tiredness

🔲 Tones the leg muscles

🔲 Stimulates the thyroid glands, fortifies the immunity

🔲 Helps women during menopause period

Head to Knee Pose

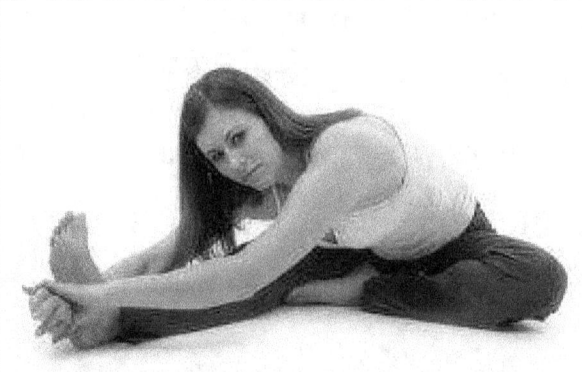

Twist your right knee and bring the right foot inside the left thigh towards your pelvis, let the right lower leg rest on the floor, try to make a right angle with the left leg.

Keep the left foot easily straight, extend the spine on an in-breath and on an out-breath turn the spine a little to face the left leg and then fold forward from the hips portion.

Keep your spine midsection open and shoulders drawn down. Now relax your face.

Stay in the posture for 2-3 minutes.

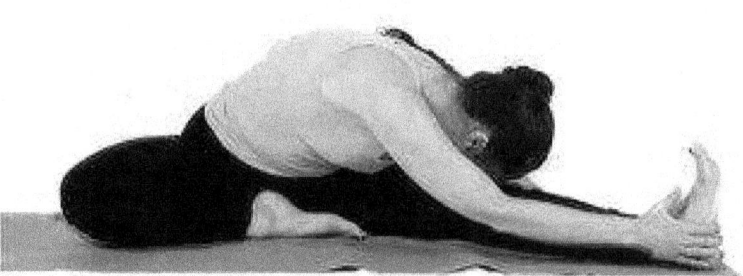

- Calms the mind and is helpful for depression

- Enhances digestion process

- Stretches the hips, back of the body and genital organs

- Relieves menstrual issues, cerebral pain, tension and weariness

- Relieves a sleeping disorder and hypertension

- Stimulates the kidneys and liver

Paschimottanasana- Seated Forward Fold

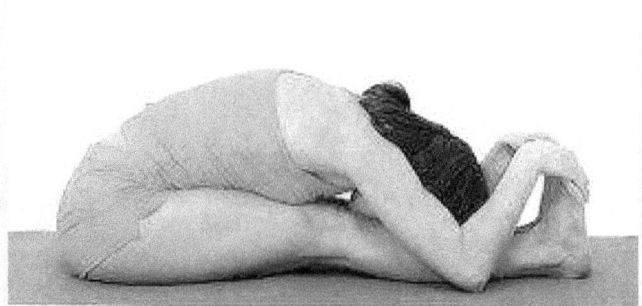

First start with exhalation and pivoting at the hips gradually brings down the midsection towards the legs. Bring the hands to the toes, feet or lower legs.

To extend the stretch- Use the arms to delicately pull the head and midsection closer to the legs. Press out through the heels and tenderly pull the toes towards you. Breathe and hold for 5-7 breaths.

To release slowly move up the spine go into normal position. Inhale in the arms over your head as you lift the torso goes into normal position.

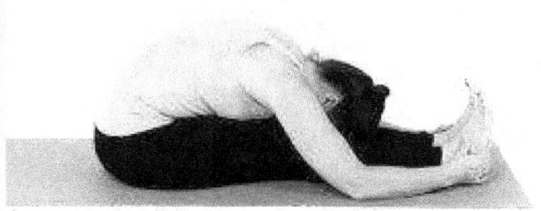

- A profound stretch for whole rear side of body from the heels to the neck

- Forward fold soothes the sensory system and emotions

- It invigorates the reproductive and urinary systems

Vajrasan- Diamond Pose

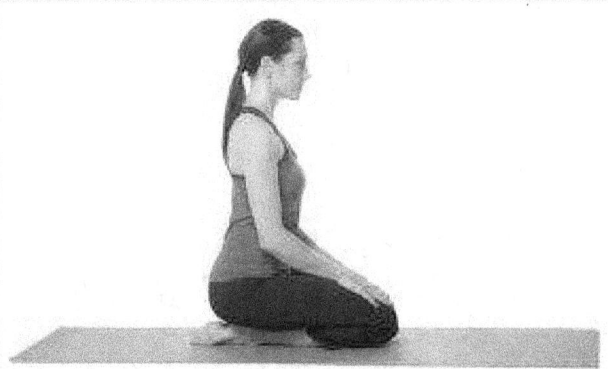

Sit on the level floor and fold your legs as demonstrated in the picture. Keep the spine erect and close the eyes. Keep the right palm on right knee and left palm on left knee.

Now begin to breathe in gradually then breathe out. When you breathe out attempt to surmise that your tensions and stresses are releasing out from your nose. Rehash these steps for 5 minutes.

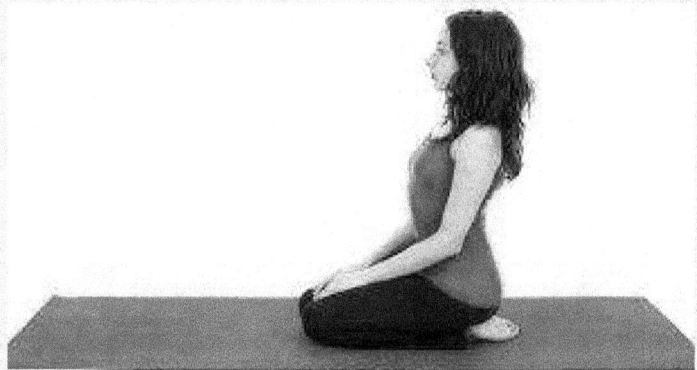

- Soothes the brain and bring balanced steadiness mind.

- Cures digestive process, constipation, gas and acidity

- Those suffering from gas issues can practice it instantly after lunch or supper

- Serves to release of back pain

- Cures stomach and urinary problems

- Reinforces the sexual organs

- Enhances blood circulation

- Serves to decrease obesity

- Reinforces the thigh muscles

- Relief the pain in arthritis patients

Pawanmuktasana- Gas Release Pose

Regular practice of Pawanmuktasana serves to fortify defecation which is exceptionally vital for evacuating waste material.

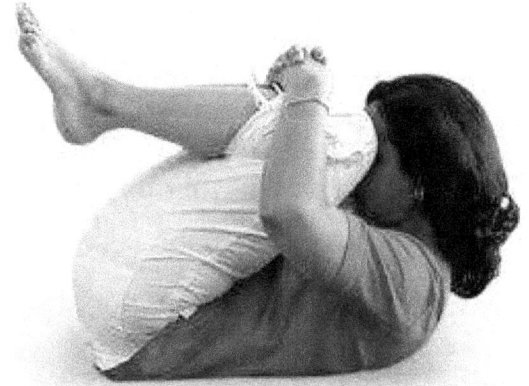

Lie level on your back and keep the legs straight and relax, breathe profoundly and systematically. Inhale gradually and lift the legs and twist in the knee.

Bring upwards to the midsection till your thigh touches to stomach, Hug your knees as shown up and lock your fingers. Try gently to touch the knee with your nose tip.

This is not simple in first time. At the same time of regular practice you can do this. Hold this position for 30 to 35 seconds.

You can progress it work 1 minute according to your capacity. Now breathe out gradually and return to the normal position.

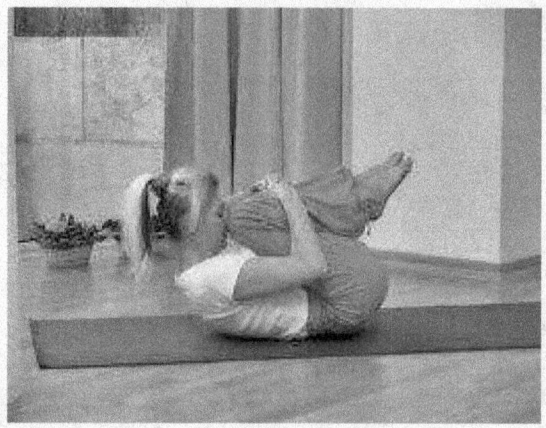

- It cures Indigestion and Constipation

- It is useful for all stomach organs

- Its consistent practice cures gastro-intestinal issues

- It is useful for stomach gas issues, acidity, joints pain, heart issues and waist pain

- It reinforces back muscle and cures back pain

- It gives level or flat stomach

- Everybody should practice this posture for level stomach

- It is exceptionally valuable for regenerative organs and for menstrual issues

Savasana- Corpse Pose

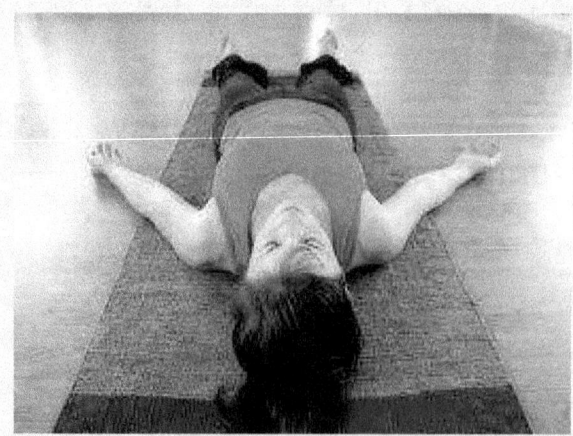

Lie level on your back, comfortably without any props or pads. Utilize little pad beneath your neck if needed. Shut your eyes. Keep your legs agreeable separated and let your feet and knees relax totally, toes confronting to the sides.

Place your arms close by, yet a bit separated from your body. Leave your palms open, confronting upward. Taking your awareness regarding distinctive body parts one by one, gradually relax your whole body.

Keep your eyes shut and take a couple of deep breaths as you bit by bit get conscious of your surroundings and the body. When you feel completely relaxed, gradually and gently open your eyes.

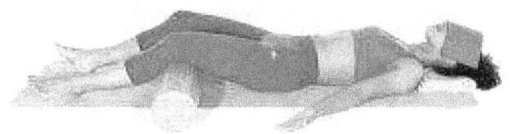

⊞ relaxes your central sensory system and calms your mind

⊞ helps soothe stress

⊞ relaxes your body

⊞ decreases beta cerebrum waves and converts to slower mind waves

⊞ reduces sleep deprivation and aides enhance your sleep

⊞ reduces migraine and tiredness

⊞ helps mitigate depression

Cat- Cow Pose

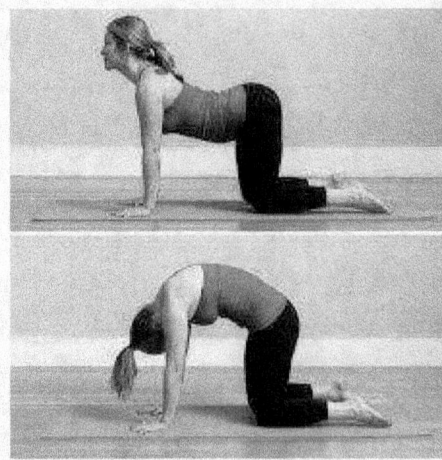

It comprises of moving the spine from a rounded position to an angled one. It's a basic movement, however one that is immensely helpful in curing back pain and keeps up a strong spine.

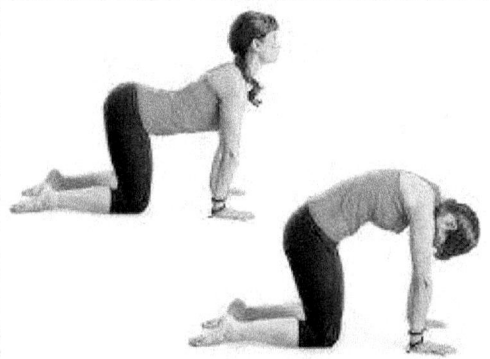

Every movement is carried out in conjunction with either an inward breath or exhalation of the breath, making this a simple exercise.

📖 It enhances spinal flexibility and natural stomach functionality

Setu-Bandhasana- Bridge Pose

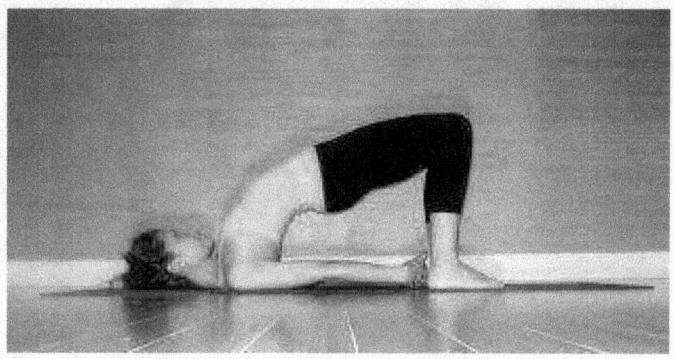

Lie level on your back with arms at your sides, palms down. Twist your knees and bring your feet level on the floor. Keep your feet hip distance separated, parallel to one another, and as near the buttock as would be prudent.

Then press your upper arms and feet into the floor and start lifting your hips towards the roof. Try to balance your weight equally within and outside of your feet.

Now move your chest towards your chin, keeping your chin lifted marginally as not to level the back of the neck. Press your tailbone in towards the pubis and move your pubis marginally towards the stomach.

With a specific end goal to hold the lower back augmented, keep the knees over the lower legs, perpendicular to the floor. Your bum ought to be firm, however not clasped.

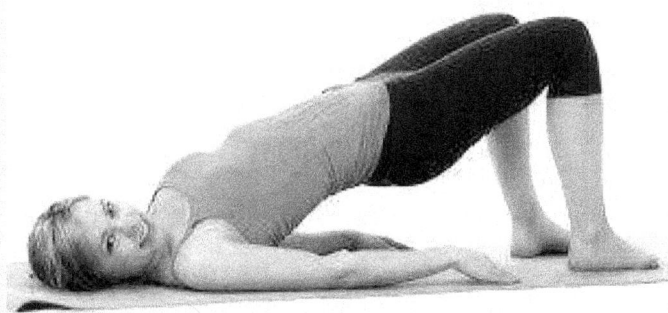

Lift your hips as high as you are capable without breaking position. In the event that you are having some difficulty holding posture, you can put your hands behind your back and press your arms into the floor, shoulder bones moved down along the spine. Hold this posture for 10 to 15 breaths.

To leave Bridge Pose, release on an exhalation, moving your spine gradually down onto the floor.

- stretches the midsection, neck, backbone, and hips

- strengthens the back, buttocks, and hamstrings

- improves circulation of blood

- helps mitigate stress and depression

- calms the mind and central sensory system

- stimulates the lungs, thyroid glands, and stomach organs

- improves digestion process

- helps alleviate symptoms of menopause

- reduces spinal pain and migraine

- reduces weariness, nervousness, and sleep deprivation

- rejuvenates tiredness

- relieves issues of asthma and HBP

Bridge posture is animating for the kidneys and henceforth mitigates the excretion system and bringing down HBP.

Practicing these specific Yoga postures, breathing has been demonstrated to have a positive impact on pulse rate. For those who've never been open to yoga previously, deep breathing can help to decrease the impacts of consistent day by day anxiety, along with the HBP.

Pranayama is a Sanskrit word and is interpreted as the Science of Breath. Pranayama can restore, revitalize and reenergize the whole body.

Conscious breathing brings down HBP (and the measure of the anxiety hormone cortisol) that is present in the body. Regular pranayama can prompt a managed lower heart beat rate.

Pranayama has been demonstrated to impact the cardiovascular system with the decrease in heart beat rate, and HBP.

Meditation is another gainful yogic practice for individuals with hypertension. The body's physical response to stress is not generally the same for everybody, except with negative stress there is no relaxation between one anxiety circumstance and the next.

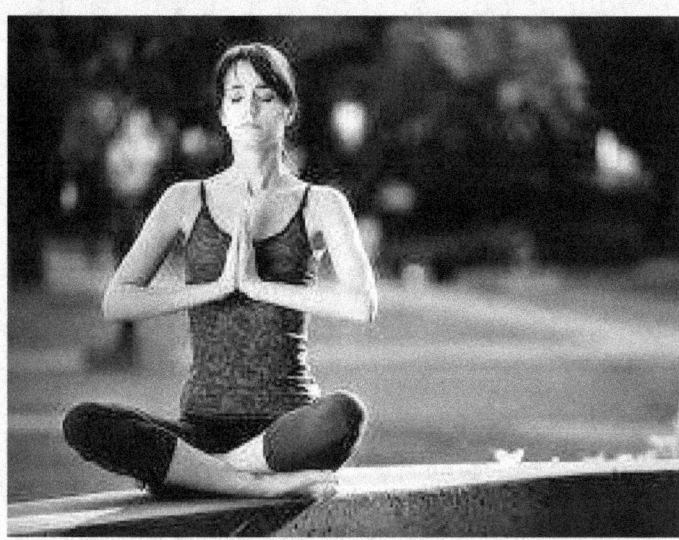

Meditation is the study of conscious awareness. The mind and body are closely associated; when the mind is totally calm, the entire body benefits complete rest.

Rehearsing meditation techniques in times of physical or mental anxiety serves to deal with the "battle or flight" reaction to negative energies and lower HBP.

When you make moves to lower HBP naturally by helping the body's own specific recuperating procedure to deal with the issue, you get Holistic healing.

Not just will you evade unwanted symptoms from HBP medicine, when pulse is brought down naturally as your sensory system gets more balanced, your entire body system benefits.

This mean you will feel better, have more vitality, will perform better all the day, and have more natural resources for adapting with stress moments.

Yoga Poses for Better Sex-Drive

Yoga is concerned on bringing the body into concordance with the mind and soul. There are studies out there that highlight how stress and poor self-perception influence your sex drive. Yoga helps us to re-interface and re-balance from within.

When you know how to take advantage of self esteem and acceptance, then our restraints appear to wash away.

Uncertainty, body insecurities, such as, considering how you are performing or what your accomplice may be thinking simply disappeared, abandoning you with bliss, sex longing, gloriousness and a wealth of astonishing times with your accomplice.

Maybe in specific way, yoga shows awareness of living just right now.

Cat-Cow Pose

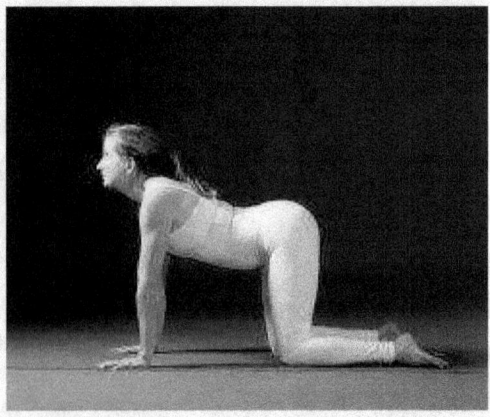 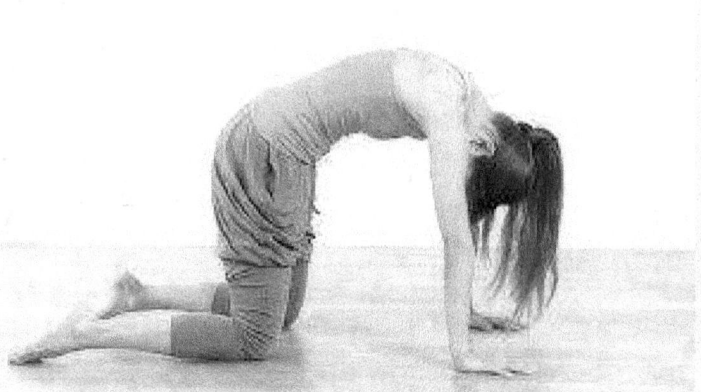

You fortify the pelvic muscles and those radiant muscles that comfort during climax as you control your tailbone of spine moving from cat to cow.

Butterfly Pose

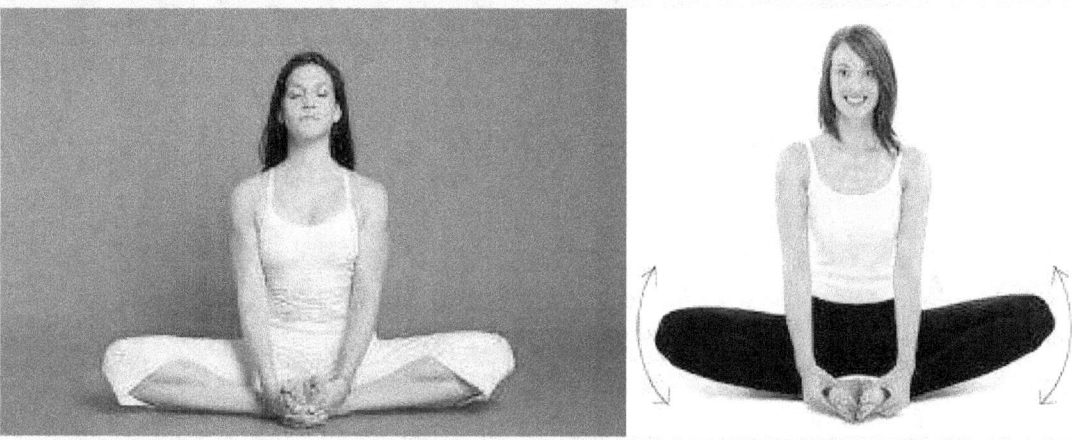

This posture and the wide-legged straddle enhanced the low sex drive. It extends the inward thighs, and opens the hips for a greater range of movement.

It enhances blood flow to the pelvic area instantly, and where the blood flows so does the vitality and essentialness. Blood circulation and accelerated blood flow are simply related to the level of arousal.

Wide-Legged Straddle Pose

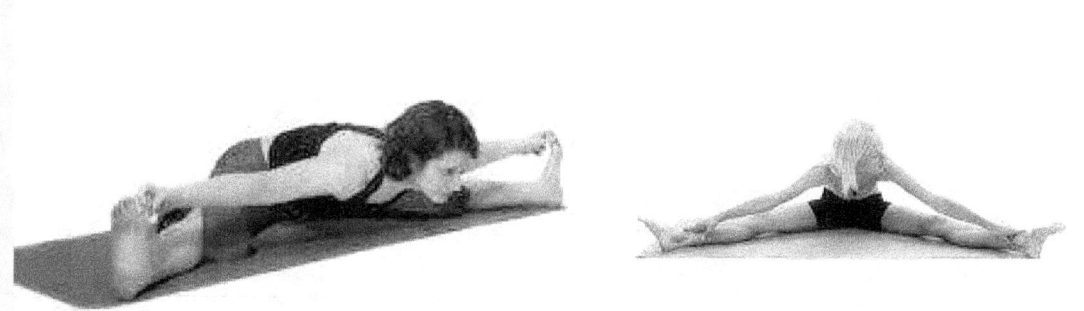

Its benefits are same as the remarkable Butterfly Pose.

Reptile/Lizard Pose

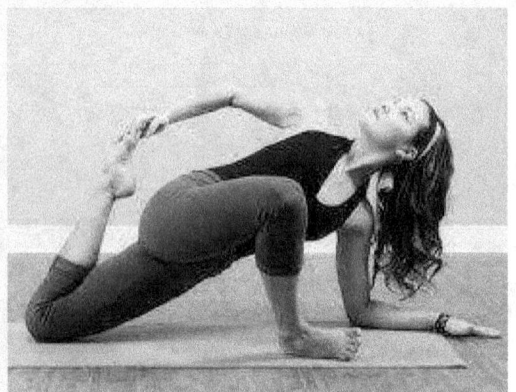 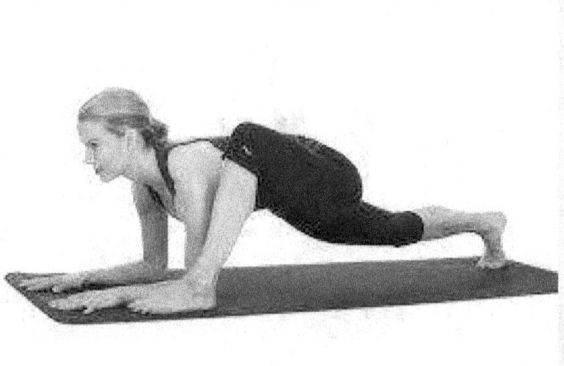

It is incredible for opening up the hips and slowing down the thinking process, making in a chilled mode.

By bringing your awareness to your breath, you move far away from your thinking process, and are brought into the present moment.

This improves your capacity to make a feeling of sexual intimacy with your accomplice.

Eagle Pose

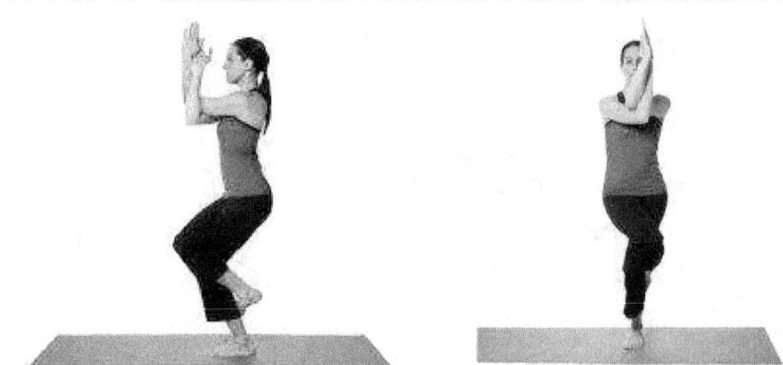

Eagle posture is so hot; it is even mentioned in the Kama Sutra. When you release the legs, the majority of the blood comes flowing through the cervix (lower part of the Uterus), which readies the entire area for some sweet sex longing!

Holding the posture itself gives a feeling of balance and steadiness quality, which is helpful if you are feeling stressed.

Your mind need to center, helping you to slow life down a bit of, permitting you to stay present and enjoy the stunning moments to take after!

Camel Pose

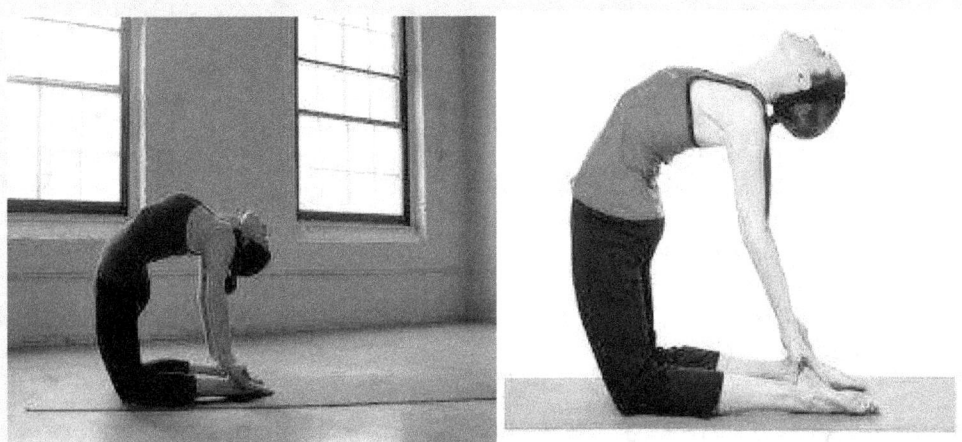

This is a heart-opening posture. Adoration, vitality and breath originate from the heart chakra. It is also extremely stimulating.

Bridge Pose

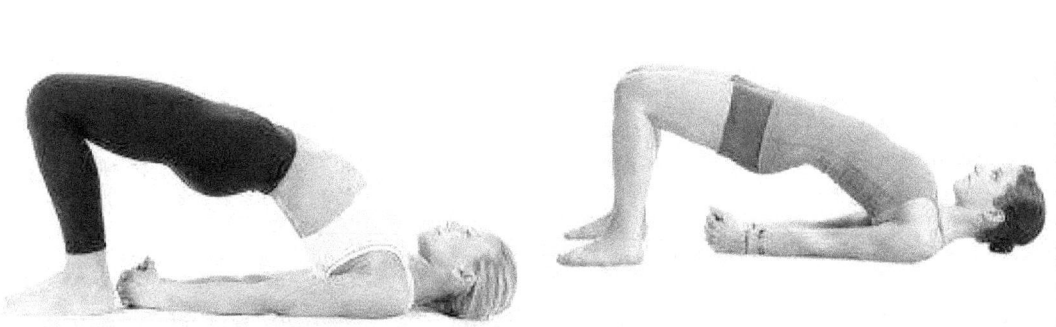

Bridge posture not just gives an exceptional hip flexor stretch; it also tones the vagina and enhances orgasms. Holding the bridge pose is same as doing pelvic muscles, because you squeeze the same pelvic muscles during sex act.

Plow Pose

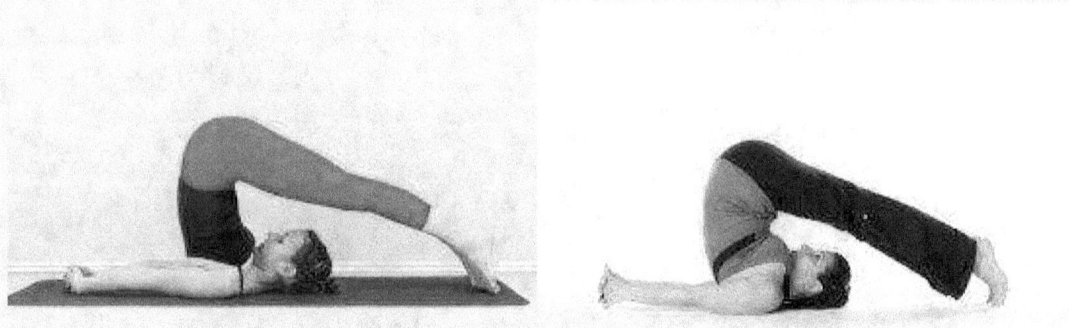

Plow permits blood to flow straight to the hips and mind that calms the brain and fortifies the body.

Likewise while you are in plow you are feeling straight toward your hips and groin and associating with that range visually, which could be a marvelous love position.

Savasana Pose

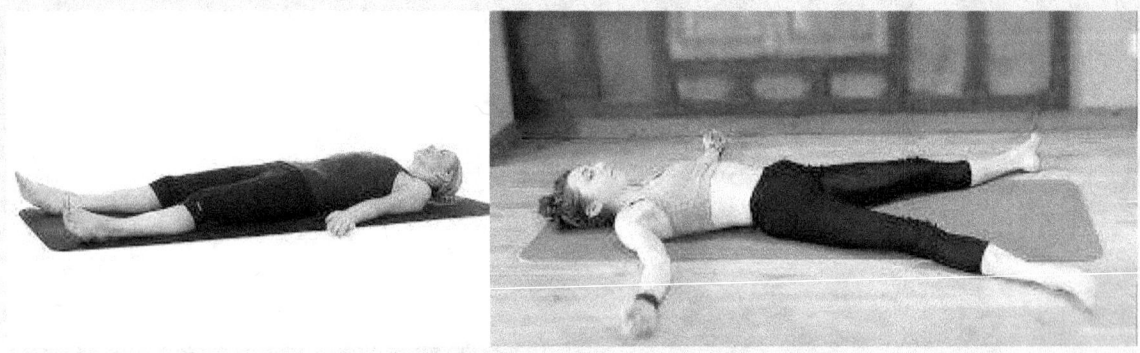

How frequently can you sit still? Sensibly! It is to assume the response is "not frequently".

Some individuals say that savasana is the hardest posture to get perfection. Most individuals consider that they can't get into their bodies.

Take a moment, and try to accomplish this posture. Anything that helps you to essentially be present in the moment is going to help you feel more arousing and sensual.

The most recognized sexual yoga postures are used to improve sexual drive and are possible anyplace in the morning. It includes contracting and relaxing the muscles of your pubic areas. You can do this 10 times, holding to a number of 5 each one time. This will help to reinforce the muscles.

Conclusion

Need to get healthy and have fabulous moments at the same time? Any of the natural activities your heart is beneficial for you, including sex act.

Sexual arousal sends the heart beat higher and the pulse rate achieves its top during climax.

Immunity

Because of sex a few progressions create in you immune system and your body generates more antibodies against diseases. Engaging in sexual relations once in a week enhances you safety against viral infections.

Self-Regard

Sex helps your respect toward oneself and confidence. After sex you feel more certain about your life stand and feel better about your autonomy. Sex makes a decent holistic union between accomplices. Having intercourse animates your mind so you feel less scared about your life issues. Sexual relations between life accomplices make their connection stronger, healthier and make their life more pleasurable.

Healthy Heart

With your increasing age your recurrence to having intercourse ought to be enhanced because of wellbeing reasons. Scientific research demonstrates that engaging in sexual relations in routine; half decreased the danger of heart attack.

Improved Stamina

By having intercourse in your schedule, stamina of your body should be progresses. During sex act it might be an advantage. For increasing in sex persistence you ought to have more sex.

It's similar to cardio respiratory activity as during sex act your muscles utilize more oxygen and your heart get to be stronger and adopts to have the capacity to pump more oxygen for body.

Options to relieve Stress

Because of having intercourse regularly your blood pressure level is kept up and you do not experience the ill effects of hypertension. Sex removes you from anxiety and brings down your pulse rate. Likewise in some individuals pulse rate drops even after the simple kissing and embracing with their accomplices.

Sound Sleep

After engaging in sex act you sleep better then without having it. Also you feel more dynamic and conscious in all the day time. All of you know for yourself how well you sleep when engaging in sexual relations. Research demonstrates that individuals engaging in sexual relations in routine don't feel troubles in sleeping.

More Calories Burned

A significant number of us practice jogging and brisk walking to burn calories. It is also the best and pleasurable approach to lose your fat.

Perhaps its not accommodating in the feeling of body workout however for an individual who having sex act actually perform full body workout and no activities can make you utilize full body muscles at the same time like this.

Sex act lasting for 60 minutes is equivalent to burning about 100 calories.

Relief of Pain

Engaging in sexual relations results a large number of improvements in your body, creating endorphins is one of them.

Because of endorphins you feel better and all the more relaxing as endorphins works adequately in decreasing pain and migraine.

Additionally sex is decent alternative for cerebral pain and provisional minor pain.

Natural healthy sex is a unique approach to help keep the body healthy and also to help keep the spirits up and feel the more emotionally connected and invigorated.

===

www.ingramcontent.com/pod-product-compliance
Lightning Source LLC
Chambersburg PA
CBHW051950280526
45789CB00009B/3239